CUT THE FAT AND LOSE THE WEIGHT...

The average American consumes a diet that contains more than 40% fats. Junk foods, fried foods, vegetable oils and shortenings are among the culprits. And the scene of the crime is your body. Not only does fat add pounds and inches, it is a well-known fact that fat increases a variety of medical risks. Keeping track of what you eat is of vital importance to both personal appearance *and* long-term health.

...THE SOLUTION:

THE FAT GRAM COUNTER
An indispensable guide to
living a healthy, low-fat life!

The COUNTDOWN TO A HEALTHIER YOU series by Berkley

THE CALCIUM AND CALORIE COUNTER
THE FAT GRAM COUNTER
THE SODIUM COUNTER

THE FAT GRAM COUNTER

Nutritional Consultant:
RANDI AARON, M.A.

Edited by
JUDITH ZIMMER

Produced by The Miller Press, Inc.

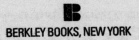

BERKLEY BOOKS, NEW YORK

THE FAT GRAM COUNTER

A Berkley Book / published by arrangement with
The Miller Press, Inc.

PRINTING HISTORY
Berkley edition / April 1986
Berkley updated and revised edition /
March 1991

ISBN: 0-425-09916-4

Contents

5

Fat Gram and Calorie Counter 33

6

Menus for Low-Fat Meals   81

FAT: WHAT IT'S ABOUT AND WHY YOU SHOULD EAT LESS OF IT

Here's a classic line:

> Why should I bother to eat this piece of cake?
> I might as well just attach it to my hip. That's
> where it's going to end up anyway.

You may laugh, but beware. There is a bit of truth here. If we do have fat deposits on our bodies (men, watch those bellies; women, those thighs), it's because we eat a fat-rich diet and consume more calories than we need to. In essence, the grams of fat in that piece of cake (or any other fatty food) do become fat deposits—if the body doesn't use those calories for energy.

The news about fat gets worse. It's a well-known fact that two of the leading causes of death in America are heart disease and cancer. And it might not be coincidental that excessive dietary fat is linked to both of these nationwide killers. Despite these findings, the average American continues to consume a diet that contains more than 40 percent fat.

Fat is everywhere—so much so that the typical American diet is a health hazard. Meats, fast food, junk foods, processed foods, fried foods and vegetable oils are among the many culprits. We eat and then wonder why we gain weight. We eat and then wonder why there are so many incidents of coronary heart disease in this country. The best reason for cutting down on the fat in your diet is, simply, good health.

Take a walk down the aisles of any supermarket. You have to steer your cart adroitly to avoid the fatty foods that surround you. Despite all the interest these days in health and nutrition, it's still hard to decipher which foods will help keep you trim and healthy.

To understand why fat is such a villain, you should know how it fits into the three basic food components. All the food we eat is either **carbohydrate, protein** or **fat**. Many of us were taught that bread, potatoes and spaghetti are fattening. It's hard to shake those old beliefs, but the truth is these **carbohydrates** are a quick energy source; they're also nutritious—if they are unrefined—and low in fat. (Unrefined foods, such as brown rice, whole wheat breads, whole wheat grains, and lentils, are full of nutrients, while refined foods, such as white bread, white rice, cookies, and cakes, have lost valuable nutrients and fiber in the refining process.)

It's not the potato itself that's fattening, it's the sour cream you may add. It's not the bread that's filled with fat, it's the butter you put on it. Compare:

Baked potato	95 calories
Baked potato with 1 tablespoon sour cream	195 calories
Slice of bread	60 calories
Slice of bread with 1 tablespoon butter	160 calories

Protein is needed for the formation of hormones and for repair and maintenance of muscles, blood, organs, skin, and hair. If you're like most Americans, you probably consume more protein than you need. Fish and chicken are good choices for protein because, unlike the most common sources—eggs, cheese, red meats—they're low in fat. For a low-fat nonanimal protein, try tofu, a fermented soybean food that looks like cheese.

Tofu has become a fairly common grocery staple in the last few years. It can be found in most supermarkets in the produce or refrigerated foods section, in any health food store, and in Oriental markets, where it is often made fresh. Tofu is an ideal diet food (and the basis for many meat-free diets) because it is high in protein and low in fat, cholesterol, and calories. Tofu is easily digestible, rich in minerals and vitamins, free of toxic chemicals, inexpensive, and easy to use. Bought fresh, it can last up to a week if you change the water it's packed in daily. It can be eaten plain with a little soy sauce and scallions, grilled, or baked in a casserole. It can even be used to make delicious, low-fat sauces and desserts.

Other soy products include imitation cheese, from Parmesan to cheddar; tempeh, a mixture of soy products and grains that makes a good meat substitute; and imitation ice cream.

Now, about **fat** . . . Fats are the most concentrated source of energy in the diet. And the most caloric. Fats contain nine calories per gram, twice the amount that carbohydrates and proteins have. Take a closer look and you'll find that not all fats are the same. There are different types of fat—from animal, vegetable, and fish sources. Each type affects the body differently.

For a long while, we've known about the link between

saturated fats and heart disease. To ward off the risk of heart disease, many people turned to polyunsaturated oils. But new research shows that an *overuse* of polyunsaturated oils could be linked to cancer. Research shows that cancer could also be caused by simply eating a diet high in overall fats.

1

YOUR NEW LOW-FAT DIET AND WHAT IT SHOULD INCLUDE

The time to start reducing your fat intake is now. The American Health Association recommends that Americans over two years of age adopt a low-fat diet. At a National Institutes of Health conference, it was determined that because of the country's high intake of calories, saturated fat and cholesterol, more than half of the population falls into the category associated with coronary heart disease.

According to research conducted by the American Heart Association, foam cells which precede the formation of fatty streaks begin to accumulate in the arteries before the age of ten and lipid-filled muscle cells develop before the age of fifteen. This evidence suggests that a low-fat diet should be required for children as well as adults, since much damage can be done to the body before the age of twenty.

Americans should reduce their total fat intake to about 30 percent or less of their total diet. (Typical fat intake for many Americans is as much as 40 to 60 percent daily.) Although the U.S. Recommended Daily Allowance for fat intake is 30 percent of the total recommended diet, many nutritionists believe that even that amount is too high and that people should strive to maintain levels less than 30 percent. Ten percent is the lowest people should go because the human body does need *some* fat. Vitamins such as A, E, D and K are fat-soluble, which means you can only absorb them if you have fat in your diet. Fats are also necessary for hormone and nerve development.

Keeping Weight Down

A high-fat diet can cause weight gain if more calories are consumed than used. You don't have to go on a diet to lose weight. Instead, nutritionists are encouraging people to build a low-fat diet into their lifestyle. At first, you might wonder how you'll be able to survive without loads of butter, cheeses and that Sunday brunch complete with eggs and bacon. But gradually you'll get used to the taste of low-fat products. They'll even make you feel more energetic, less sluggish. You might just get so used to eating them that fatty foods will begin to become unappealing.

A low-fat diet and even moderating excess will help you lose or maintain weight. You'll be fit and trim and lean because you'll be cutting down on a hefty supply of calories. (Remember each gram of fat contains nine calories—twice as many as carbohydrates or proteins.) Think of it this way: say you're a woman trying to take in about 1500 calories a day. One tablespoon of fat provides about 100 calories. That tablespoon alone is a little less than 15 percent of your day's intake. Instead of using one tablespoon of butter on your bread, try apple butter with 37 calories a tablespoon and no fat. You'll be able to fulfill that 1500-calorie requirement and eat substantial meals if you replace some of the fat in your diet with carbohydrates. The bottom line with fat is that the calories really add up.

Tracking Down Dietary Fat

Most of us don't realize the amount of fat that is in what we eat. For example, nuts, avocados and olives are all rich in fat. And there is a certain amount of fat that lurks in even the most unsuspected of foods, such as vegetable oils, grains, nuts, crackers, fish, chicken, and desserts. Even if you don't eat any *added* fats, you'll consume some fat from these unsuspected sources. According to Jane Brody in *Jane Brody's Nutrition Book:* "Your daily need is for a mere tablespoon of dietary fat to maintain good nutrition. Yet the average American adult consumes six to eight tablespoons of fat a day."

How Much Fat Should You Consume?

New findings indicate that Americans ought to revise the balance of dietary fats consumed in order to ward off the risk of cancer and heart disease. You should:

1. Reduce total fat intake to 30 percent or less.
2. Cut out as many saturated fats as you can or eliminate them entirely.
3. Achieve a balance between polyunsaturates and monounsaturates.

Experiment to see how low your daily intake of fat can go: Start at Level 1 and try to work your way down to Level 3, eliminating all saturates.

	Saturates	Polyunsaturates	Monounsaturates
Level 1	10 percent	10 percent	10 percent
Level 2	2 percent	8 percent	8 percent
Level 3	None	10 percent	10 percent

"So what do I eat?" you might ask. If you reduce your fat intake, but then consume empty non-nutritious calories from sources such as white breads and sweets, you won't see one of the primary benefits of a low-fat diet—namely, weight loss. *Take up the slack of calories with complex carbohydrates*. Complex carbohydrates are high in fiber and fiber is known to prevent cancer and reduce levels of triglycerides and cholesterol.

You should consume the following carbohydrates:

- Fresh fruits and vegetables, including lentils, legumes, peas
- Whole grains, including whole wheat breads, whole wheat cereals, brown rice, barley, corn, buckwheat, millet, oats, popcorn.

2

THE DIFFERENT TYPES OF FAT AND WHAT THEY DO TO YOU

Not too long ago, scientists thought that all calories were created equal. In the laboratory, it was assumed that the calories in a serving of chocolate ice cream were the same as an equal number of calories in a bowl of whole wheat pasta. In other words, one would need to expend X amount of energy to burn the number of calories contained in either the ice cream or the pasta. On the basis of new metabolic research conducted by Dr. Martin Katahn, author of the book, *The T-Factor Diet*, and other scientists around the country, we learn that when you eat a calorie of fat (butter, ice cream, fried food, sauces, etc.) it is quickly and easily stored in fat cells—and inevitably shows up on our thighs, stomachs, and rear ends. However, when a calorie of complex carbohydrate is consumed (whole grain bread, fish, apple, pasta, for examples) the body must exert more effort to get energy, or make fat, from that calorie. A lot of the value of that calorie is eliminated as heat. This is what Dr. Katahn has named the "T-Factor," or thermogenic effect. Thus, it is the fat in your diet that determines the fat on your physique. The best dieting trick of all is to reduce the number of fat calories you consume, and eat mostly protein and car-

SATURATED FAT

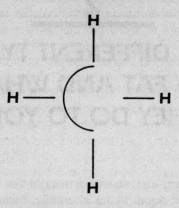

MONOUNSATURATED FAT

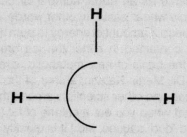

POLYUNSATURATED FAT

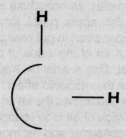

bohydrate calories—you don't even have to worry too much about how *many* of those calories you eat. It's also important to know that not all *fats* are created equal.

Fats are divided into two groups: saturates and unsaturates. Their difference lies in the chemistry of the molecules. To understand why fats are dense heavy molecules which have almost twice as many grams per calorie as carbohydrates, compare the chemical design of each. Carbohydrates are complex sugar molecules with water (hydrogen and oxygen) added to carbon. Fats, on the other hand, have only hydrogen added to them.

When all the hydrogen slots are filled, the fat is called saturated. When hydrogen slots are left empty, the fat or oil is said to be unsaturated. *Mono*unsaturated fat has a single slot open; *poly*unsaturated has several left open. (The accompanying illustration depicts the chemical structure of saturated animal fats and the unsaturated vegetable fats, monounsaturated and polyunsaturated.) The more open positions there are, the more likely it is that the fat will be liquid at room temperature. In fact, room temperature can be used as a means for determining types of fat: saturated fats (from animal sources) are always solid at room temperature (except for coconut and palm oils), polyunsaturated fats (vegetable sources) are always liquid at room temperature, and monounsaturated fats (vegetable sources) are usually liquid at room temperature.

Saturated Fats

Sources: *Red meat, dairy products including hard cheeses, whole milk and whole milk products, eggs, coconut and palm oil*

You can see from its chemical structure that saturated fats are the densest of all the fat molecules. We've known for a long time that saturated fats are unhealthy. Eating too much can lead to the buildup of fatty deposits along the walls of the blood vessels or arteries, which in turn prohibit the circulation of blood. This buildup of fatty deposits is linked to coronary heart disease and atherosclerosis, a condition where fats clog the arteries.

There are two types of harmful fats associated with heart disease: triglycerides and cholesterol. When stored within the body, fat is called a triglyceride: fat chains are attached in sets of three to a compound called glycerol. Increased blood-triglyceride levels cause red blood cells to clump together, decreasing blood circulation and oxygen transport.

The other deposit material is cholesterol, a waxy, fatlike substance found within the body. A certain amount of cholesterol is needed for the body to function properly—specifically, to form body tissue and produce sex and adrenal (nervous system) hormones. An extremely low level of cholesterol is an indication of malnutrition.

High levels of cholesterol in the blood contribute to heart and blood disease. The body produces some cholesterol on its own. But in most cases it is a diet high in saturated fats and cholesterol which causes blood cholesterol to reach levels associated with heart disease.

Cholesterol is carried through the body by lipoproteins (or fatty proteins) which are formed in the liver. There are two kinds of lipoproteins: HDL or high-density lipoproteins and LDL or low-density lipoproteins. The HDL are "good" because they don't cause atherosclerosis, instead they remove cholesterol from artery walls. The LDL does the opposite; it keeps cholesterol in the blood. Because you can't get rid of the LDLs completely (everyone has a certain amount of both types), the goal is to have a good ratio of HDL to LDL. It has been found that people with coronary heart disease have a high level of LDL.

A low-fat diet promotes the formation of HDL and can help you to maintain a healthy ratio of HDL to LDL. People who are on a low-fat diet and *exercise* usually have higher levels of HDL. Experts believe that *aerobic exercise* can help protect you from heart disease.

Exercise—in which you get your heart rate up and keep it there for an extended period of time—is the best, safest way to get excess body fat off and keep it off. Aerobic exercise has come a long way since the early 80's when we were told to "go for the burn." Many shin splints, wrecked knees, and bad backs later, kinesiologists decided that it's not necessary to work so *hard* to burn body fat—instead you can go for longer periods of lower-intensity exercise, and significantly reduce the incidence of injury. That activity doesn't have to be very vigorous, it can be brisk walking, bicycling, rowing, or dancing. Stationary bicycles, rowing machines, and cross-country training machines are all good alternatives to more stressful high-impact aerobics, jumping jacks, running, or jogging. Take it easy, but move continuously for at *least* twenty-five minutes—forty minutes is ideal. The point of aerobic exercise is to get your heart rate up and make your metabolism work harder than usual to start burning fat. And one of your goals when exercising should be to enjoy what you're doing, to ensure that you'll keep at it. Tennis, paddle ball, racket ball, gymnastics, running or jogging, badminton, basketball, soccer, and swimming are just a few good aerobic activities that will keep you interested in the exercise.

On page 97 you'll find a list of current exercise videos that feature a thirty minute or more aerobic workout with stretches, exercises, and routines that are fun and safe.

Another recent advance in exercise physiology is the recognition of the role that muscle-building plays in reducing fat. Research has shown that larger muscles need more energy to function; so, the larger the muscles, the more calories the body will burn, even when inactive. By lifting free weights or using the Nautilus machines at the gym, reducing the number of fatty calories consumed and increasing the number of carbohydrate calories, you can build muscle and trim fat. Pounds and inches will disappear, and a stronger, healthier body can be shaped in weeks by working out only three times a week.

Polyunsaturated Fats

Sources: *vegetable oils, including safflower, corn, and linseed*

When it became known that saturated fats were associated with high cholesterol levels, people were encouraged to turn to vegetable fats. They did so with enthusiasm, believing that they could ward off heart disease, reduce cholesterol levels and, at the same time, still enjoy tasty fats. So polyunsaturates took the limelight.

Cancer producing?

Researchers believe that a diet high in overall fat is linked to cancer—particularly, cancer of the breast and cancer of the colon, two of the most common cancers in the U.S. But because so many people turned to polyunsaturates in hopes of reducing heart disease, experts now believe that we *overdid* it on the polyunsaturates.

They've discovered that vegetable oils taken from plants are not as wholesome as they were once thought to be. Remember that when an oil is taken from inside a vegetable, it is an unsaturated carbon chain and it has several empty spaces. When these oils are heated, they become less healthy for you. The empty spaces within the polyunsaturates fill up with oxygen. This process, known as oxidation, makes the oil rancid and turns it into a toxic compound known as trans-fatty acids. (Remember, since polyunsaturates have more open spaces than monounsaturates, this process is much more likely to occur with polyunsaturates.)

The breakdown of this rancid fat inside the body produces substances known as "free radicals." These are chemically reactive molecules which are unstable and unhealthy. Your body handles a certain amount of these every day because some are necessary for metabolic reactions; in these circumstances, the free radicals don't do any damage because the body supplies enzymes which control them. Too large a quantity of polyunsaturated fats or oils tends to increase the formation of free radicals, accelerating the aging process and destroying healthy tissue.

The more polyunsaturates you consume, the more free radicals are formed inside the body. The National Cancer Institute and the American Heart Association recommend that we eat less polyunsaturated fats and balance our intake of all monounsaturated, polyunsaturated, and saturated fats. Our bodies make a certain amount of saturated and monounsaturated fats by themselves, but they don't produce any polyunsaturates—in particular, the essential fatty acid known as linoleic acid. So a small amount of polyunsaturates is necessary to a healthy diet. The healthiest way to consume polyunsaturated oils is cold, as in salad dressings.

A replacement for saturates?

A careful look at the polyunsaturates on the market today reveals that all polyunsaturates are not processed the same way. Take margarine, for example. It was designed as a substitute for butter, a highly saturated source of animal fat. Your margarine stick might say that it's of vegetable origin, but look closely at the small print. Some brands are "hydrogenated," which means that the vegetable oil has been altered. It has been "saturated" with hydrogen to make it hard. (You can tell that margarine sticks are not purely unsaturated because they are hard.) People think they are doing themselves a big favor by eating margarine instead of butter. Although margarine is healthier than butter because it doesn't have any cholesterol, both butter and margarine have the same number of calories.

Look at labels closely: many processed foods, including such grocery items as crackers and whole wheat breads, are "hydrogenated" or "partially hydrogenated." This means that they contain a form of vegetable fat that is similar to saturated fat.

Tropical oils such as palm, coconut, and palm kernel are highly saturated oils and the least healthy of all vegetable fats. They are also cheaper to use in processed foods which is why you'll find them regularly on the labels of processed cakes, cookies, and candy bars. They are also found in dairy substitutes: imitation cream cheese, whipped cream and dessert toppings, coffee cream substitute, and artificial sour cream. Although in recent years food ingredient labeling has become more specific, often tropical oils may be called simply "vegetable oil" on the package. The danger of highly saturated fats like tropical oil is that our bodies make cholesterol more easily from them than from the monounsaturated or polyunsaturated fats.

Monounsaturates

Sources: *Olive oil, peanut oil, nuts*

The focus has shifted from one extreme to the other, from the most saturated fats to the most unsaturated. We were once told to eat polyunsaturates and now we're told not to. Now attention is turning to the middle, the monounsaturates, which are not as unsaturated as polyunsaturates and are therefore not a suspect for cancer-producing free radicals.

For a long time, it was believed that the monounsaturated fats were neutral in their effects on blood cholesterol; they didn't raise it, didn't lower it. But new findings at the Texas Health Science Center and elsewhere show that monounsaturated fat is more effective than polyunsaturated in lowering cholesterol and reducing the risk of heart disease.

Although both polyunsaturates and monounsaturates reduce cholesterol, monounsaturates do a better job of it. Here's why: They both lower levels of bad cholesterol, LDL, but polyunsaturates also lower the good cholesterol, HDL. Monounsaturates, on the other hand, don't change the HDL levels, according to reports in *The Journal of Lipid Research.*

Researchers are also hopeful that safflower and sunflower oils, which are high in polyunsaturates, can be reformed to produce monounsaturated oils.

A ten-year, seven-country study conducted at the University of Minnesota has observed the link between fat in diet and coronary heart disease. The Finns, with Americans following a close second, consumed the most fat including saturated fats and had the highest blood cholesterol levels. The Japanese, who ate more polyunsaturated fats, had low cholesterol levels and rare incidences of heart disease deaths. The Greeks and Italians had almost no heart disease deaths and most consumed olive oil, a monounsaturate.

The time is right for monounsaturates. Make olive oil a household staple. Especially use it for cooking, since it is more stable than polyunsaturates when heated.

Fish Oils

In the past, fish oil was thought to be fuel for the brain and bad for the heart because of high cholesterol levels. But now scientists know more. They believe that fish oils are one of the healthiest sources of fat we can eat because they are protective; they can actually lower harmful fat deposits and cholesterol in the blood. The discovery came after researchers observed that Greenland Eskimos who eat lots of fat have low levels of coronary heart disease. The important clue was that they also subsist on fish.

Fish oils are polyunsaturated fats, even though they don't come from vegetable sources. There are two such fatty acids: eicosapentaenoic acid, or EPA; and docosahexaenoic acid, or DHA. Together they are known as the omega-3 long-chain fatty acids. Most fish and shellfish contain them, but the oilier, fattier fish are the heartiest source. Although experts at Oregon Health Sciences University in Portland who conduct omega-3 research say the studies are still inconclusive, it is believed that these acids are protective, lowering triglycerides and cholesterol and also reducing clogging within the artery walls.

Fish-oil supplements (MaxEPA) and cod liver oil (lower in value than MaxEPA) have also become popular at some health food stores. But because findings are inconclusive, supplements are not recommended. Too much fish oil could cause damage. Experts recommend that, instead, you get fish oil from the fish itself, eating a varied amount of lean or fatty fishes and shellfish several times a week. (Supplements in moderation could be helpful if you can't eat fish.) Fatty fishes include tuna, mackerel, salmon, bluefish, sardines, mullet, rainbow trout, lake trout, herring, sablefish and shad. (Read the labels on canned tuna and salmon carefully. Some are packed in vegetable oils. A positive alternative are those packed in water.) Keep in mind that breaded fishes, fried fish, and fish in cream sauces have added fat content. Broiled, baked, poached, or steamed fish is the best bet for a nutritious meal.

3

HOW TO REDUCE THE AMOUNT OF FAT IN YOUR DIET

The best way to reduce fat is to simply stop eating it. But fat is everywhere, in all different kinds of foods. By becoming aware of fat and the foods which are high in fat, you'll have a fighting chance at reducing your intake.

Hidden Fats

Reducing fat can be difficult because there is so much hidden in our diets. When counting your fat calories per day, use the following values as guidelines to estimate the amount of fat used in prepared foods.

Vegetables and salads
- ½ teaspoon fat per ½ cup of "buttered" or stir-fried vegetables
- At least 1 teaspoon of fat for 10 small french fries
- 1 tablespoon of fat for potato salad, cole slaw, tuna or chicken salad

Entrees
- ½ teaspoon fat per ounce of pan-fried or basted meat, fish or poultry
- 1 teaspoon fat per ounce of breaded and fried meat, fish or poultry
- About 1 teaspoon fat per fried egg

Gravy and sauces
- 1 teaspoon for every 2 tablespoons of gravy or cream sauce

Breads
- 1 teaspoon for each small muffin, biscuit, pancake, waffle or cornbread (and that's before you *add* the butter)

Eating at home
Here are ways to reduce the amount of fat you consume at home:
- Cut down on the amount of processed and packaged foods you eat. Read labels. Be on the lookout for added hydrogenated fats or lard.
- Cut out added fats such as mayonnaise or creamy dressings. Lemon, spices, or a sprinkle of grated parmesan cheese (1 tablespoon equals only 33 calories) can replace cream sauces for flavoring. Apple butter (made from the fruit and cider without sugar) or unsweetened preserves for toast are better than butter.

Cooking

Following are some ways to cut down on the amount of fats used in cooking. (For more information, see chapter 4, *Substitutions*.)

- If you must eat red meat, then choose lean cuts and reduce portion size to about 4 ounces of cooked meat. Trim fat from meat and remove skin from poultry before cooking, if you can. Brown meats by broiling.
- Chill soups and stews to remove congealed fat (you'll save 100 calories per tablespoon).
- Make use of herbs and spices. Vinegar, mustard, tomato juice and bouillon can be used as seasonings instead of butter and sauces.
- Start cutting back by ⅓ or ½ the fat required by recipes. If a casserole calls for 6 tablespoons, use 3 or 4. If a muffin recipe suggests 1 cup of oil, try ¾. If that works, use only ⅔ next time. With packaged rice mixes, you can usually omit butter or margarine without changing the taste.
- When sautéing vegetables, cut the amount of oil recommended in half or leave it out completely and add water or broth. Then steam.
- If you find your foods lose moisture without fat, use broth, skim milk, wine, or fruit juice for extra flavor.
- Use no-stick pans or a lecithin spray like PAM or Mazola No-stick, to cook anything from pancakes to meat without using any fat at all.

Dining Out

Most restaurants these days—four-star establishments, diners, and even fast food places—try to accommodate the dieter or the person on a restricted diet. You can get a salad at McDonald's or Burger King (but beware of the dressings, you're better off not using any at all), a diet plate of cottage cheese and fruit at any diner, a plate of broiled fish and vegetables (or a variety of "spa cuisine" choices) at a fine restaurant. If you are determined to avoid fat, and assertive enough, you don't need to consume hidden fats or sugars when dining out.

You *do* have control over what you're served at a restaurant. Take charge of the situation before you even arrive at the restaurant. Call and inquire about food preparation or ask if special requests are honored. The New York Heart Association suggests you ask the restaurant whether they do, or would on request:

1. Serve margarine (rather than butter) with the meal?
2. Serve skim (rather than whole) milk?
3. Prepare a dish using vegetable oil or olive oil rather than butter?
4. Trim visible fat off meat or skin poultry?
5. Boil, bake, steam, or poach (rather than sauté or deep-fry) meat, fish, or poultry?
6. Limit portion size to 4 to 6 ounces of cooked meat, fish or poultry?
7. Serve butter, gravy, or sauce on the side?

Do anything you can to ensure that you don't get more fat than you want. Order as it suits you: choose appetizers as a main portion or order à la carte.

When ordering from the menu, *look for* the following terms. They indicate low-fat preparation:

steamed, roasted, broiled, poached, in its own juice, tomato juice, garden fresh, dry broiled (in lemon juice or wine)

Avoid foods described as:

buttery, buttered, in butter sauce, sautéed, fried, pan-fried, crispy, creamed, cream sauce, in its own gravy, au gratin, hollandaise, parmesan, in cheese sauce, marinated (in oil), stewed, basted, casserole, pot pie

The Low-Fat Dos and Don'ts of Menu Reading

Appetizers

DO CHOOSE: steamed seafood, raw or steamed vegetables, fresh melon, or other fruit

AVOID: buttery crackers, regular cheeses, cream soups

Bread

DO CHOOSE: bread or breadsticks, whole wheat if possible

AVOID: spreads or margarine, garlic bread or buttered breads

Entrees

DO CHOOSE: poultry, fish, or shellfish (because they can be prepared without added fat)

AVOID: broiled entrees (which are sometimes basted in fat)

Salads

DO CHOOSE: fresh greens like lettuce or spinach, vegetables like cucumbers, radishes, tomatoes, carrots, and onions

AVOID: cheese, eggs, meat, or bacon (watch for rich dressings), chef and Caesar salads

Side Dishes

DO CHOOSE: vegetables cooked fat-free (boiled or steamed), rice, baked potato, or any other grain

Desserts

DO CHOOSE: fresh fruit, fruit ices, sherbets, gelatin, or angel food cake

Eating Ethnic

Just because you're going the low-fat route doesn't mean you have to give up your favorite ethnic foods. Learn how to detect the low-fat selections on the menu.

Italian

Stick to vegetable soups like minestrone and pasta dishes with tomato sauces (like marinara) or wine-based sauces (like Marsala). Stay away from cream or cheese sauces; they're fattening. Seafood selections are always a good choice; try steamed mussels or a combined platter like linguine with red clam sauce.

French

La cuisine française is known for its richness and fattening ingredients such as butter, cream, and eggs. Instead of cream sauces like béchamel or béarnaise, order dishes prepared in wine sauces such as brodelaise. Patés are very fattening, as is another French favorite, duck. But if you stick to simple dishes, such as steamed mussels or oysters with a salad or cooked vegetables, you'll be able to have a low-fat meal and still enjoy the flavor of France. Try a fresh fruit sorbet for dessert.

Chinese

Make a meal out of steamed dim sum (dumplings stuffed with fish, meat, or vegetable). Go for the fish or vegetable fillings. Try steamed or boiled vegetable dishes with chicken or fish. Beware of dishes with "egg" contents, such as egg drop soup, since they'll increase your cholesterol level. Avoid fried or deep-fried dishes and heavy sauces like shrimp and lobster sauce. Ask for brown rice instead of white.

Mexican

This could almost be easy. Mexican food has lots of selections that can fit into your low-fat diet. Stay clear of melted cheeses, guacamole. But try any variety of chicken, chilis, rice, beans (if they're not prepared in lard), and tortillas. Instead of fried tortilla chips, ask if baked or soft tortilla chips are available.

Japanese

A variety of seafood, chicken, and noodle dishes await you. Try dishes made with tofu. Sashimi—raw fish and rice wrapped in seaweed—is another good choice, as is tekka maki roll, kappa maki roll or California roll. Tempura dishes have been deep-fried in batter, so steer clear of them.

4

SUBSTITUTIONS: GETTING RID OF FAT AND EATING WELL

The key to reducing fat in cooking (or just plain snacking) is to substitute a less fatty food for a fatty one.

Avoid	Replace With
Animal fats	Polyunsaturated oils
Butter, 1 cup	Margarine, 1 cup or better: ⅞ cup of polyunsaturated or olive oil
Sour cream	Yogurt
Meat in recipes	Tofu cubes, cooked legumes or vegetables (chick peas, lentils, kidney beans), cooked grains (bulgur, rice, noodles)
Ricotta cheese, sour cream	Low-fat cottage cheese, part skim ricotta, low-fat yogurt
Mayonnaise	Yogurt
Cheddar cheese, 1 oz.	Low-fat cheese, 1 oz.
Cheddar cheese, 1 cup	Grated parmesan cheese or low-fat cheese, 2 T.

Avoid	Replace With
Cream	Evaporated milk
Egg, 1 whole	Egg whites, 2
Ice cream	Ice milk, frozen yogurt, tofutti, frozen fruit bars, sorbets
Junk food	Fresh fruit, bagels, crackers without hydrogenated fats or lard, cereals, air-popped popcorn, whole wheat pretzels, unroasted nuts and seeds

Liquid Diets

While many people may lose huge amounts of weight quickly on these diets of 400 to 800 calories per day, the pounds will come back almost certainly, along with damage to one's metabolism and muscle tissues.

The problem with such low calorie diets is that when the body is so severely deprived of a sensible number of calories per day, the metabolism—a very delicate mechanism—switches into its starvation prevention mode and slows down drastically in order to create energy by storing fat. So what starts out to be a weight loss program quickly becomes a fat conservation dilemma as your body reacts to the starvation level of daily caloric intake. If, after losing pounds on the liquid diet, you want to start eating even moderate amounts of food, you will gain weight because your metabolism is not prepared to burn calories efficiently.

You cannot take shortcuts when trying to lose weight sensibly and successfully. You need to exercise daily, build calorie-burning muscle, reduce the amount of fat in your diet, and ear regular, balanced, *small* meals.

Liquid diets, or any other diet that delivers starvation levels of calories to your body, will end up thwarting any long-term weight loss or maintenance programs by upsetting the balance of your metabolism.

5

FAT GRAM AND CALORIE COUNTER

Let this book help you in your fight against fat. Keep track of the amount of fatty foods you buy and how much fat you eat. Check the following 1000 food listings to make sure you're not letting fat calories get the better of you.

Each entry lists the food item, the amount, the number of calories, and the amount of fat, in grams. Foods that contain predominantly one type of fat are indicated by either *s* (saturated fat), *m* (monounsaturated fat) or *p* (polyunsaturated fat). At the end of most categories there is a note on the category's general type(s) of fat.

To determine the percentage of fat in your daily diet, add up the total grams of fat per day, multiply by 9 (number of calories per gram of fat), divide by the total number of calories consumed and multiply by 100.

For example: Item	5 fat grams
Item	10 fat grams
Item	20 fat grams
Total	35 fat grams

35 fat grams × 9 = 315 calories

(If you are a woman, you should eat approximately 1500 to 1800 calories per day; if you are a man, 1800 to 2000.)

If you eat 1500 calories a day, 315 calories of which is fat here is how you would calculate the percentage of fat in your diet:

$$\frac{315}{1500} \times 100 = x\%.$$

$$x = 21\%$$

(Use the same formula to determine percentage of polyunsaturated, monounsaturated or saturated fat in your daily diet.)

Calories and Fat Gram Counts

BEVERAGES

	Amount	Calories	Fat Grams
ALCOHOLIC			
Beer	12 oz.	148	—
Beer, light	12 oz.	100	—
Eggnog	4 oz.	335	15.8 *s*
Gin, rum, vodka, whisky			
80 proof	1 oz.	65	—
90 proof	1 oz.	74	—
100 proof	1 oz.	83	—
Martini	3½ oz.	140	—
Wine			
Champagne	4 oz.	84	—
Dessert, sweet	3½ oz.	153	—
Sherry	2 oz.	84	—

	Amount	Calories	Fat Grams
Table, red	3½ oz.	76	—
Table, white	3½ oz.	80	—

JUICES: FRUITS/VEGETABLE

	Amount	Calories	Fat Grams
Apple (bottled)	8 oz.	116	.3
Carrot	8 oz.	96	.2
Cranberry cocktail (bottled)	8 oz.	147	.1
Grape (bottled)	8 oz.	155	.2
Grapefruit			
Fresh	8 oz.	96	.3
Canned	8 oz.	93	.2
Frozen	8 oz.	102	.3
Orange juice			
Fresh	8 oz.	111	.5
Canned	8 oz.	104	.4
Frozen	8 oz.	112	.1
Orange/grapefruit (frozen)	8 oz.	101	.1
Pineapple	8 oz.	139	.2
Tomato	8 oz.	41	.2
V-8	8 oz.	53	.1
Prune	8 oz.	181	.1

LOW-CALORIE SODA

	Amount	Calories	Fat Grams
Diet Coke	12 oz.	1	—
Diet Pepsi	12 oz.	1	—
Diet Seven-up	12 oz.	4	—
Tab	12 oz.	1	—

With soda, any diet type is better—just compare!

NONALCOHOLIC

	Amount	Calories	Fat Grams
Coffee	6 oz.	3	trace
Tea	8 oz.	0	—

BEVERAGES

	Amount	Calories	Fat Grams
PUNCHES, JUICE DRINKS			
Gatorade	8 oz.	39	—
Hawaiian Punch	8 oz.	120	trace
Lemonade (frozen)	8 oz.	94	trace
Tang, grape	6 oz.	89	—
orange	6 oz.	89	—
SODA			
Coca-Cola	12 oz.	144	—
Ginger ale	12 oz.	133	—
Root beer	12 oz.	163	—
Seven-up	12 oz.	144	—

CANDY & CANDY BARS

	Amount	Calories	Fat Grams
Almond Joy	1 oz.	151	7.8 s
Butterscotch	6 pieces	116	2.5 s
Caramels	3 pieces	112	2.9 s
Choc.-cov. almonds	1 oz.	159	12.2 s
Choc. kisses	6 pieces	154	9.0 s
Fudge, choc.	1 oz.	112	3.4 s
Fudge, choc. w/nuts	1 oz.	119	4.9 s
Gum drops	28 pieces	97	.2
Hard candy	6 pieces	108	.3
Hershey's Special Dark	1.02 oz.	157	8.6 s
Hershey's milk choc.	1.02 oz.	160	9.4 s
Jelly beans	10 pieces	66	0.0

	Amount	Calories	Fat Grams
Life savers	5 pieces	39	.1
M&M's	1.69 oz. pkg.	220	10.0 s
Marshmallows	1 lg. pkg.	25	0.0
Mints, small	14 pieces	104	.6
Nestlé Crunch	1.06 oz.	160	8.0 s
Oh Henry	1 oz.	139	7.1
Peanut brittle	1 oz.	123	4.4 s

COMBINATION FOODS (Entrees & Frozen Foods)

	Amount	Calories	Fat Grams
Beans & franks, in tomato sauce, canned	7¾ oz.	332	14.5
Beans, refried, w/sausage, canned	½ cup	194	13.0
Beef Oriental, in sauce w/ veg. & rice	9⅛ oz.	280	9.0
Beef pie, frozen	8 oz.	409	20.0
Beef veg. stew	1 cup	218	10.5
Chicken a la King, canned	5¼ oz.	180	12.0
Chicken a la King, frozen	8 oz.	220	9.0
Chicken a la King, w/rice, frozen	9½ oz	330	11.0
Chicken & rice	7 oz.	234	12.6
Chicken fricassee	7 oz.	328	18.6
Chicken, fried, w/whipped potatoes	7¼ oz.	410	23.0
Chicken Parmigiana	7 oz.	308	14.8
Chicken pie, frozen	10 oz.	500	28.0

COMBINATION FOODS

	Amount	Calories	Fat Grams
Chicken pie	4 oz.	273	15.7
Chili Con Carne, w/ beans, canned	7¾ oz.	305	15.0
Chili, meatless, canned	½ cup	190	7.0
Chili, w/franks, canned	1 cup	320	17.0
Chow mein, chicken, frozen	8 oz.	86	1.6
Enchiladas, beef & cheese, w/gravy, frozen	8 oz.	280	13.6
Fish creole, homemade	3½ oz.	86	2.7
Fritter, corn	3½ oz.	377	21.5
Frozen Breakfasts			
French toast & sausage	4½ oz.	300	17.0
Pancakes & sausage	6 oz.	500	25.0
Frozen Dinners			
Beans & Franks	11¼ oz.	550	19.0
Beef	11 oz.	290	10.0
Chicken, fried, breast	11 oz.	590	31.0
Chicken, fried, 3-course	15 oz.	630	31.0
Chop suey	12 oz.	282	8.2
Chow mein, chicken	12 oz.	282	8.5
Enchilada, beef	12 oz.	479	17.3
cheese	12 oz.	459	16.7
Fish	8¾ oz.	382	14.6
Fish & chips	10¼ oz.	450	22.0
Ham	10 oz.	380	13.0
Macaroni & beef	12 oz.	400	15.0
Macaroni & cheese	12½ oz.	390	14.0
Meatloaf	19 oz.	916	57.7
Mexican	16 oz.	608	25.4
Ocean perch	8¾ oz.	434	17.6
Pepper oriental	11 oz.	349	7.3

	Amount	Calories	Fat Grams
Pork loin	11¼ oz.	470	22.0
Salisbury steak	11 oz.	390	24.6
Sirloin, chopped	10 oz.	460	25.0
Spaghetti & meatballs	11½ oz.	450	15.3
Turkey	11½ oz.	360	11.0
Veal parmigiana,			
w/tomato sauce	8 oz.	391	21.8
Green pepper, stuffed			
w/beef, breadcrumbs	1	315	9.0
w/beef and sauce	6½ oz.	190	9.0
Hash, corned beef, canned	3½ oz.	184	12.5
Lasagna			
cheese, frozen	8 oz.	300	12.0
w/meat, frozen	8 oz.	300	14.0
zucchini, frozen	11 oz.	260	6.0
Macaroni & beef, tomato			
sauce, canned	7½ oz.	220	8.0
boil-in-bag	9 oz.	240	7.4
Macaroni & cheese, canned	7⅜ oz.	170	6.0
frozen	8 oz.	282	12.0
Pizza			
Cheese, frozen	¼ pie	320	12.8
Cheese	1 slice	153	5.4
Deluxe, frozen	¼ pie	367	18.6
Pepperoni	¼ pie	356	18.2
Sausage, frozen	¼ pie	375	19.5
Ravioli, beef in sauce, frozen	1 ravioli	60	2.0
Sandwiches			
Bacon, let., tom., mayo.,			
white bread	1	282	15.6
Chicken, let., mayo., white			
bread	1	303	14.4

COMBINATION FOODS

	Amount	Calories	Fat Grams
Chicken salad, white bread	1	245	8.6
Club	1	590	20.8
Corned beef, rye	1	296	10.8
Cream cheese, jelly, white bread	1	368	16.0
Egg salad, white bread	1	279	12.5
Ham & mayo., white bread	1	281	15.4
Frank (hot dog)	1	260	15.2
Peanut butter, jelly, white bread	1	374	15.1
Peanut butter, jelly, whole wheat bread	1	385	15.2
Roast beef, mayo., white bread	1	328	22.6
Roast beef & gravy, white bread	1	429	24.5
Roast pork & mayo., white bread	1	288	14.7
Tuna salad, white bread	1	278	14.2
Turkey & mayo., white bread	1	402	18.4
Scallops, oriental & veg., w/rice, frozen	11 oz.	230	2.0
Spaghetti & meat sauce, canned	7½ oz.	230	10.0
homemade	10 oz.	396	20.7
Spaghetti & tomato sauce, w/meatballs, canned	7⅜ oz.	210	8.0
w/meatballs	3½ oz.	134	4.7
Spaghetti & franks, tomato sauce, canned	7⅜ oz.	210	10.0

	Amount	Calories	Fat Grams
Steak & green peppers, frozen	8 oz.	190	8.0
Sweet & Sour pork	7 oz.	386	21.7
Turkey a la King	6 oz.	212	11.7
Turkey pie, frozen	8 oz.	460	25.0
Veal scallopini	4 oz.	199	11.3

Most of these combination foods are high in saturated fat and/or hydrogenated fats.

DAIRY PRODUCTS

	Amount	Calories	Fat Grams
MILK			
Whole (3.7%)	1 cup	157	8.9
Skim	1 cup	86	0.4
Low-fat (2.0%)	1 cup	121	4.7
Low-fat (1.0%)	1 cup	102	2.6
Evaporated, whole, canned	1 oz.	42	2.4
skim, canned	1 oz.	25	.1
Soybean milk	1 cup	87	4.0
Soybean milk powder	1 oz.	120	5.7
Buttermilk, cultured	1 cup	99	2.2
Buttermilk, dry	1 T	25	.4
MILK BEVERAGES			
Chocolate milk			
1% fat (low-fat)	1 cup	158	2.5
whole	1 cup	208	8.5
Hot choc. (whole milk)	1 cup	218	9.1

DAIRY PRODUCTS

	Amount	Calories	Fat Grams
Eggnog, nonalcoholic	1 cup	342	19.0
Instant breakfast, vanilla, w/whole milk	1 cup	280	8.0
Milkshake, chocolate	1 avg.	356	8.1
vanilla	1 avg.	350	9.5

MILK PRODUCTS
Cheeses

	Amount	Calories	Fat Grams
Blue	1 oz.	100	8.2
Brie	1 oz.	95	7.9
Camembert	1 oz.	85	6.9
Cheddar	1 oz.	114	9.4
Cheddar, grated	1 cup	455	37.5
Cottage cheese, creamed	1 cup	217	9.5
Cottage cheese, low-fat 1%	1 cup	164	2.3
Cottage cheese, low-fat 2%	1 cup	203	4.4
Cream cheese	1 oz.	99	9.9
Edam	1 oz.	101	7.9
Feta	1 oz.	75	6.0
Gouda	1 oz.	101	7.8
Gruyere	1 oz.	117	9.2
Limburger	1 oz.	93	7.7
Mozzarella	1 oz.	80	6.1
Mozzarella, part skim	1 oz.	72	4.5
Muenster	1 oz.	104	8.5
Parmesan, grated	1 T	33	1.5
Parmesan, hard	1 oz.	111	7.3
Provolone	1 oz.	100	7.6
Ricotta, part skim	½ cup	171	9.8
Ricotta, whole	½ cup	216	16.1

	Amount	Calories	Fat Grams
Romano	1 oz.	110	7.6
Swiss	1 oz.	107	7.8
Cheese food			
American	1 oz.	93	7.0
Smoked	1 oz.	91	6.7
Swiss	1 oz.	92	6.3
Cheese Pastuerized/			
Processed American	1 oz.	106	8.9
Swiss	1 oz.	95	7.09
Cheese spread			
American	1 oz.	82	6.0
Cheese products			
Cheese fondue	¼ cup	170	11.7
Cream & Whipped Toppings			
Half & half	1 T	20	1.7
Light	1 T	29	2.9
Sour cream	1 T	26	2.5
Whipping, heavy	1 T	52	5.6
Whipping, light	1 T	44	4.6
Frozen, Cool Whip	1 T	13	1.0
Cream Substitutes			
Liquid/frozen	½ oz.	20	1.5
Powdered	1 T	11	.7
Yogurt			
Low-fat, plain	1 cup	144	3.5
Low-fat, coffee, vanilla	1 cup	197	2.8
Low-fat, fruit	1 cup	225	2.6
Whole milk, plain	1 cup	139	7.4

Whole-milk dairy products, including cheeses, are high in saturated fats. Low-fat dairy products have a reduced amount of saturated fat, while skim-milk products have virtually no fat.

DESSERTS

	Amount	Calories	Fat Grams
BROWNIES			
Butterscotch	1	115	5.0
Choc., w/nuts & icing	1	81	3.5
CAKES			
Angel food	1 piece	161	.1
Apple streusel crumb	1 piece	200	8.3
Banana, Sara Lee	1/8 cake	175	6.9
Black Forest, Sara Lee	1/8 cake	194	9.3
Boston cream pie	1 piece	332	10.3
Carrot	1 piece	249	12.0
Cheesecake	1 piece	257	16.3
Cheesecake, strawberry, Sara Lee	1/6 cake	222	8.2
Choc., mix	1/12 cake	250	11.0
Choc., devil's food w/choc. icing	1 piece	233	10.8
Choc. fudge, w/vanilla icing, mix	1/6 cake	280	10.0
Coconut, Sara Lee	1/2 cake	246	13.1
Fruit cake, dark	1 piece	152	6.1
German choc., Pepperidge Farm	1 piece	297	16.0
Marble, w/white icing, mix	1 piece	165	4.3
Pineapple upside-down	1 piece	236	9.1
Pound, Sara Lee	1/10 cake	125	6.9
Shortcake w/strawberries	1 serving	344	8.9
Sponge	1 piece	188	3.1
Yellow	1 piece	283	12.4

	Amount	Calories	Fat Grams
COOKIES			
Animal	15	120	2.9
Capri, Pepperidge Farm	1	82	4.6
Chocolate	1	93	3.3
Choc. chip	1	46	2.7
Fig bars	1	53	1.0
Gingersnaps	1	34	1.6
Graham cracker, choc.-covered	1	62	3.1
Granola, Pepperidge Farm	2	318	15.4
Macaroons	1	67	3.2
Oatmeal	1	80	3.2
Oatmeal raisin	1	61	2.6
Peanut	1	57	2.3
Shortbread	1	42	2.3
Sugar	1	89	3.4
Sugar wafers	2	53	2.1
Vanilla, creme sandwich	1	69	3.1
Vanilla wafers	3	51	1.8
CUSTARD			
Homemade	½ cup	153	7.3
Packaged mix	½ cup	161	5.4
Banana	½ cup	143	4.6
Chocolate	½ cup	144	4.4
Vanilla	½ cup	143	4.6
DANISH			
Apple	1	121	4.9
Cheese	1	131	7.2
Plain	1	161	8.8

DESSERTS

	Amount	Calories	Fat Grams
DOUGHNUTS			
Cake	1	105	5.8
Cake, w/sugar icing	1	151	6.5
Creme-filled	1	122	4.7
Jelly	1	226	8.8
FROZEN YOGURT			
Danny on a stick	1	65	1.0
Danny on a stick, choc./carob coated	1	135	7.5
Danny-yo	½ cup	110	1.0
Fruit varieties	½ cup	108	1.0
Tofutti, hard pack	4 oz.	210	7 g
GELATIN			
All flavors	½ cup	81	trace
Low-cal, D-Zerta	½ cup	8	trace
ICE CREAM			
Chocolate	1 cup	295	16.0
French vanilla, soft	1 cup	377	22.5
Strawberry	1 cup	250	12.0
Vanilla, (10% fat)	1 cup	269	14.3
Vanilla, (16% fat)	1 cup	349	23.7
Cremesicle	1	103	3.1
Ice cream sandwich	1	167	6.2
Ice cream bar, vanilla, w/choc. coating	1	162	10.6
Popsicle	1	65	0.0

	Amount	Calories	Fat Grams
ICE-MILK			
Chocolate	2/3 cup	137	4.6
Strawberry	2/3 cup	133	3.1
Vanilla	1 cup	184	5.6
ICES			
Lime/orange	1 cup	247	trace
PASTRY			
Creme puff, w/custard filling	1	245	14.6
Eclair, w/choc. icing & custard filling	1	316	15.4
PIES			
Apple crisp	1/2 cup	302	8.1
Apple	1/8 pie	282	11.9
Banana cream, frozen	1/8 pie	240	12.0
Blueberry	1 piece	387	17.3
Cherry, frozen	1/8 pie	400	16.0
Choc. cream	1/8 pie	301	17.3
Coconut custard, frozen	1/8 pie	330	15.0
Lemon meringue, frozen	1/8 pie	310	10.0
Mince meat, frozen	1/8 pie	252	9.6
Peach cobbler	1/3 cup	160	6.4
Peach crisp	1/2 cup	249	9.3
Peach, frozen	1/8 pie	365	16.0
Pecan	1 piece	334	18.3
Pumpkin	1 piece	317	16.8
Shoofly	1 piece	441	16.4
Strawberry	1 piece	228	9.1
Sweet potato	1 piece	342	18.2

DESSERTS

	Amount	Calories	Fat Grams
PUDDINGS			
Banana cream, mix	1/2 cup	172	4.3
Bavarian chocolate	1 serving	347	24.9
Bread w/raisin	3/4 cup	314	10.0
Butterscotch	1/2 cup	207	4.7
low-cal.	1/2 cup	69	.2
Chocolate, mix	1/2 cup	179	4.5
Lemon, mix	1/2 cup	178	4.3
Rice, canned	2/5 cup	115	3.0
Tapioca	1/2 cup	133	5.0
Vanilla, mix, skim milk	1/2 cup	147	.3
Vanilla, mix, whole milk	1/2 cup	177	4.3
Vanilla, mix, low-cal.	1/2 cup	71	.2
PUDDING POPS			
Chocolate	1	99	2.7
Vanilla	1	93	2.6
SYRUPS			
Choc. fudge topping	2 T	97	3.8
Chocolate syrup	2 T	73	.4
Walnut, in syrup	3 T	169	1.3

Dessert foods are made with saturated and/or hydrogenated fats with the exception of those made with skim milk, low-fat yogurts, ices, and gelatins.

EGGS

	Amount	Calories	Fat Grams
Boiled	1 large	79	5.6
Fried	1 large	83	6.4
Omelet, plain	1 large	95	7.1
Poached	1 large	79	5.6
Scrambled w/milk	1 large	95	7.1
White	1 large	16	trace
Yolk	1 large	63	5.6
Duck egg	1 large	130	9.6
Goose egg	1 large	267	19.1
Quail egg	1 large	14	1.0

EGG DISHES
Crepes
	Amount	Calories	Fat Grams
Apple, frozen	1	195	5.0
Chicken, continental, frozen	2	320	15.0
Ham & veg., frozen	2	305	16.0
Quiche, Florentine, frozen	9½ oz.	625	34.0
Quiche, Lorraine, frozen	9½ oz.	720	41.0

Souffle
	Amount	Calories	Fat Grams
Cheese, homemade	4 oz.	240	18.8
Spinach, frozen	⅖ cup	116	6.8

EGG SUBSTITUTES
	Amount	Calories	Fat Grams
Frozen	¼ cup	96	6.7
Liquid	1½ oz.	40	1.6
Powdered	.35 oz.	44	1.3
Country Morning	½ cup	173	12.1

EGGS

	Amount	Calories	Fat Grams
Egg Beaters	¼ cup	30	0.0
Egg Replacer	1 oz.	95	trace
Scrambled Land o' Lakes	½ cup	143	9.1

All eggs and egg dishes are high in saturated fats, with the exception of egg white and quail eggs.

FAST FOOD

	Amount	Calories	Fat Grams
ARBY'S			
Club sandwich	1 serving	560	30.0
Ham & cheese sandwich	1 serving	380	17.0
Roast beef sandwich	1 serving	350	15.0
Roast beef and cheese	1 serving	450	22.0
Turkey	1 serving	510	24.0
ARTHUR TREACHER'S			
Chicken, fried	1 serving	364	21.6
Chips	1 serving	275	13.1
Coleslaw	1 serving	118	8.0
Fish chowder	1 serving	112	5.4
Fish, fried	1 serving	354	19.7
Krunch pup (hot dog)	1 serving	204	14.9
BURGER KING			
Cheeseburger	1 serving	350	17.0
French fries	1 serving	210	11.0
Hamburger	1 serving	290	13.0

	Amount	Calories	Fat Grams
Hamburger, whopper	1 serving	630	36.0
Whopper w/cheese	1 serving	740	45.0
Whopper, Double-beef	1 serving	850	52.0
Onion rings	1 serving	270	16.0
Shake, chocolate	1 serving	340	10.0
Shake, vanilla	1 serving	340	11.0

KENTUCKY-FRIED CHICKEN
Chicken, fried

	Amount	Calories	Fat Grams
Drumstick, extra crispy	1 serving	155	9.0
Drumstick, original recipe	1 serving	117	6.5
Side breast, extra crispy	1 serving	286	17.8
Side breast, original	1 serving	199	11.7
Wing, extra crispy	1 serving	201	13.5
Wing, original	1 serving	136	9.0
Coleslaw	1 serving	121	7.5
Corn on the cob	1 serving	169	2.8
French fries	1 serving	184	6.7
Gravy	1 serving	23	1.8
Mashed potatoes	1 serving	64	.9

McDONALD'S

	Amount	Calories	Fat Grams
Egg McMuffin	1 serving	327	14.8
English muffin w/butter	1 serving	186	5.3
Hot cakes w/butter, syrup	1 serving	500	10.3
Sausage, pork	1 serving	206	18.6
Scrambled eggs	1 serving	180	13.0
Big Mac	1 serving	563	33.0
Cheeseburger	1 serving	307	14.1
Chicken McNuggets	6	314	19.0
Fillet-o-fish	1 serving	432	25.0
French fries	1 serving	220	11.5
Hamburger	1 serving	255	9.8

FAST FOOD

	Amount	Calories	Fat Grams
Quarter-pounder	1 serving	424	21.7
Quarter-pounder w/cheese	1 serving	524	30.7
Cookies, McDonaldland	1 serving	308	10.8
Pie, apple	1 serving	253	14.3
Pie, cherry	1 serving	260	13.6
Shake, chocolate	1 serving	383	9.0
Shake, strawberry	1 serving	362	8.7
Shake, vanilla	1 serving	352	8.4
Sundae, hot fudge	1 serving	310	10.8

PIZZA

	Amount	Calories	Fat Grams
Cheese, reg. crust of 12" pizza	½	653	12.4
Cheese, thin crust of 10" pizza	½	359	9.8

SUBMARINES

	Amount	Calories	Fat Grams
Ham, salami, cheese	8"	639	23.4
Roast beef	8"	611	22.5
Tuna	8"	685	33.6

TACO BELL

	Amount	Calories	Fat Grams
Burrito, bean	1 serving	350	10.8
Burrito, beef	1 serving	466	21.0
Enrichito	1 serving	373	16.9
Frijoles & cheese	1 serving	232	6.0
Taco	1 serving	162	8.6
Tostada	1 serving	179	6.0

WENDY'S

	Amount	Calories	Fat Grams
Cheeseburger	1 serving	580	34.0

	Amount	Calories	Fat Grams
Chili con carne	1 serving	230	8.0
French fries	1 serving	330	16.0
Hamburger	1 serving	470	26.0
Shake, chocolate	1 serving	390	16.0

Most fast foods are high in saturated and/or hydrogenated fats.

FATS, SHORTENINGS AND OILS

	Amount	Calories	Fat Grams
Butter	1 t	36	4.1 *s*
Butter, whipped	1 t	27	3.1 *s*
Butterbuds, liquid	2 t	12	0.0
Margarine, corn	1 t	34	3.8 *p*
Margarine, imitation, corn	1 t	17	1.9 *p*
Mayonnaise	1 t	99	11.0
Mayonnaise, imitation, soybean	1 t	35	2.9 *p*

Even though margarines are made with polyunsaturated fats, they are hydrogenated in the process. Mayonnaise is made with a combination of saturated and polyunsaturated fats.

ANIMAL

	Amount	Calories	Fat Grams
Bacon fat	1 T	126	14.0 *s*
Chicken fat	1 T	115	12.8 *s*
Pork fat, lard	1 T	116	12.8 *s*

SHORTENINGS

	Amount	Calories	Fat Grams
Crisco	1 T	106	12.0 *s*

FATS, SHORTENINGS AND OILS

	Amount	Calories	Fat Grams
Soybean and palm	1 T	113	12.8 s
Lard and veg. oil	1 T	115	12.8 s

OILS

	Amount	Calories	Fat Grams
Coconut	1 T	120	13.6 s
Corn	1 T	120	13.6 p
Cottonseed	1 T	120	13.6 p
Olive	1 T	119	13.5 m
Palm	1 T	120	13.6 s
Peanut	1 T	119	13.5 m
Puritan	1 T	124	14.0 p
Safflower	1 T	120	13.6 p
Sesame	1 T	120	13.6 p
Soybean	1 T	120	13.6 p
Sunflower	1 T	120	13.6 p

FISH, SHELLFISH AND SEAFOOD

	Amount	Calories	Fat Grams
Abalone, raw	3½ oz.	98	.5
Anchovy, canned	3 fillets	21	1.2
Bass, striped, broiled	3½ oz.	228	12.8
Bluefish, broiled	½ fish	192	6.3
Caviar, granular	1 t	26	1.5
Clams, soft (meat)	41 g.	82	1.9
Cod, broiled	3½ oz.	162	5.0
Crab cake	1 oz.	46	2.5
Crab, steamed	3½ oz.	93	1.9

	Amount	Calories	Fat Grams
Crayfish, raw	3½ oz.	72	.5
Fishcakes, fried	3½ oz.	172	8.0
Fish fillet			
batter-dipped, frozen	6 oz.	440	31.0 s
light & crispy, frozen	4 oz.	311	23.0 s
Fish sticks, frozen	4½ sticks	176	8.9
Flounder, baked	3½ oz.	202	8.2
Haddock			
broiled	3½ oz.	141	6.6
fried	3½ oz.	165	6.4
Halibut broiled	3½ oz.	214	8.8
Herring, Atlantic, broiled canned, tomato sauce, smoked, kippered	3½ oz.	211	12.9
Lobster	1 lb.	413	8.6
Lobster Newburg	7 oz.	388	21.2 s
Lobster thermidor	5½ oz.	405	26.6 s
Mackerel, Atlantic, canned	½ cup	192	11.7
Pacific, canned	3½ oz.	180	10.0
Oysters, canned	3½ oz.	76	2.2
raw	5-8 med.	66	1.8
Perch	1 lb.	431	11.3
Salmon, red, canned	⅖ cup	171	9.3
broiled, baked	3½ oz.	182	7.4
smoked	3½ oz.	176	9.3
Sardines, canned, in oil	8	311	24.4
in tomato sauce	1 can	230	17.0
Scallops, steamed	3½ oz.	112	1.4
Shrimp	3½ oz.	91	.8
Shrimp, canned, dry	3½ oz.	116	1.1
Smelt	4-5 med.	200	13.5
Sole	1 fillet	80	.8

FISH, SHELLFISH AND SEAFOOD

	Amount	Calories	Fat Grams
Swordfish, broiled	3½ oz.	174	6.0
Trout	3½ oz.	196	11.2
Tuna, canned			
in oil	6½ oz.	381	19.9
canned, in water	6½ oz.	237	3.5
Tuna salad	½ cup	170	10.5 s
White fish, smoked	3½ oz.	155	7.3

Fish and seafood are a source of all three types of fat. Fatty fishes are an especially good source of EPA oils and are lower in saturated fat than red meat.

FRUITS

	Amount	Calories	Fat Grams
Apples, medium	1 serving	81	.5
dried	10	155	.2
Applesauce, sweetened	½ cup	97	.2
unsweetened	½ cup	53	.1
Apricots, raw	3 med.	51	.4
canned, heavy syrup	4 halves	75	.1
canned, water pack	4 halves	20	trace
dried	1 med.	83	.2
Banana	1 med.	105	.6
Blackberries, raw	½ cup	37	.3
frozen, unsweetened	1 cup	97	.7
Blueberries	1 cup	82	.6
Boysenberries, frozen,			
unsweetened	1 cup	66	.4

	Amount	Calories	Fat Grams
Cantaloupe	1/2 melon	94	.74
Cherries, raw	10	49	.7
Cranberry sauce, jellied, canned	1/2 cup	209	.2
Dates, dried	10	228	.4
Figs, dried	10	447	2.2
Fruit cocktail, canned			
heavy syrup	1/2 cup	93	.1
juice packed	1/2 cup	56	trace
water packed	1/2 cup	40	.1
Grapefruit, pink	1/2 med.	37	.1
white	1/2 med.	39	.1
Grapes, American	1 cup	58	.3
European	1 cup	114	.9
Honeydew melon	1/4 small	33	.3
Kiwi fruit, raw	1 med.	46	.3
Lemon	1 med.	17	.2
Lime	1 med.	20	.1
Mango, raw	1 med.	135	.6
Orange, naval, raw	1 med.	65	.1
Papaya, raw	1 med.	117	.4
Peach, raw	1 med.	37	.1
canned, heavy syrup	1 cup	190	.3
dried	10 halves	311	1.0
Persimmon, raw	1 med.	32	.1
Japanese, raw	1 med.	118	.3
Pineapple, raw	1 cup	77	.7
canned, heavy syrup	1 cup	199	.3
canned, juice packed	1 cup	150	.2
Plantain, cooked	1 cup	179	.3
Plum, raw	1 med.	36	.4
Prunes, dried	10	201	.4

FRUITS

	Amount	Calories	Fat Grams
Quince, raw	1 med.	53	.1
Raisins	2/3 cup	300	.5
Raspberries, raw	1 cup	61	.7
frozen, sweetened	2/5 cup	103	.2
Strawberries, raw	1 cup	45	.6
frozen, sweetened	1 cup	52	.2
Tangelos	1 med.	39	.1
Tangerines	1 med.	37	.2
Watermelon	1 cup	50	.7

GRAIN PRODUCTS

	Amount	Calories	Fat Grams
BREAD			
Bagel	1	163	1.4
Biscuit, mix	1	93	3.1
Cornbread, whole ground	2″ sq.	93	3.2
Cracked wheat	1 slice	66	.9
Italian, enriched	1 slice	55	.2
Matzo	1 piece	117	.3
Mixed grain	1 slice	64	.9
Oat bran bread (all natural)	1 slice	65	—
Raisin	1 slice	70	1.0
Pita, whole wheat	1 slice	140	2.0
Pumpernickel	1 slice	79	.4
Rye	1 slice	56	.3
Sourdough	1 slice	68	.5
White	1 slice	64	.9
Whole wheat	1 slice	61	1.1

	Amount	Calories	Fat Grams
Bread crumbs	1 cup	345	40.0
Breadsticks	1 reg.	23	.2
Muffins			
English	1	135	1.1
Blueberry	1	126	4.3
Bran	1	112	5.2
Corn, w/enriched cornmeal	1	141	4.5
Whole wheat	1	103	1.1
Rolls			
Brown 'n' serve	1	92	2.2
Buttermilk	2	168	5.0 s
Croissant	1	108	6.1 s
Dinner	1	85	2.1
French, enriched	1	137	.4
Hamburger, hot dog	1	114	2.1
Raisin	1	165	1.7
Rye	1	55	1.6
Sandwich	1	162	3.1
White, enriched, hard	1	88	1.7
Whole wheat	1	90	1.0
French toast, frozen	2 slices	170	4.3
homemade	1 slice	153	6.7
Pancakes, plain	3 med.	210	1.6
buckwheat	1 med.	90	4.1
Waffles, homemade	1 large	245	12.6*
frozen	1 med.	95	3.2

CEREAL, COOKED

	Amount	Calories	Fat Grams
Cream of rice	¾ cup	95	.1

*usually made with butter, eggs or margarine

GRAIN PRODUCTS

	Amount	Calories	Fat Grams
Cream of wheat	¾ cup	100	.4
Cream of wheat, instant	¾ cup	115	.4
Farina	¾ cup	87	.1
Maypo	¾ cup	128	1.8
McCann's Irish Oatmeal	⅓ cup	100	2
Oats, reg./quick	¾ cup	108	1.8
Oats, instant	1 pack	104	1.7
Roman Meal	¾ cup	111	.7
Wheatena	¾ cup	101	.8
Whole wheat, hot, natural cereal	¾ cup	113	.7

CEREAL, READY-TO-EAT

	Amount	Calories	Fat Grams
All Bran	⅓ cup	71	.5
Alpen	1 oz.	110	5.0
Bran 100%	½ cup	76	1.4
Bran Buds	⅓ cup	73	.7
Bran Flakes 40%	⅔ cup	93	.5
Cap'n Crunch	¾ cup	119	2.6
Cheerios	1¼ cup	111	1.8
Corn Flakes	1¼	110	.1
Crispix	1 cup	110	—
Fruit Loops	1 cup	111	.5
Fruit 'n' Fibre, w/apples, cinnamon	½ cup	87	.3
Granola	⅓ cup	126	4.9
Grapenuts	¼ cup	101	.1
Life	⅔ cup	104	.5
Nutra-grain, barley	¾ cup	106	.2
corn	⅔ cup	108	.7
rye	¾ cup	102	.2
wheat	¾ cup	102	.3

	Amount	Calories	Fat Grams
Product 19	¾ cup	108	.2
Puffed rice	1 cup	57	.1
Puffed wheat	1 cup	52	.2
Quaker 100% Natural	¼ cup	133	6.1 *s*
Raisin Bran, Kellogg's	¾ cup	115	.7
Rice Krispies	1 cup	112	.2
Shredded Wheat	1 biscuit	83	.3
Special K	1⅓ cup	111	.1
Sugar-Frosted Flakes	¾ cup	108	.1
Total	1 cup	100	.6
Wheat Chex	⅔ cup	104	.7
Wheat germ, toasted	¼ cup	108	3.0
Wheaties	1 cup	99	.5

CRACKERS

	Amount	Calories	Fat Grams
Cheese	5	81	4.9 *s*
Cheese w/peanut butter	1.5 oz.	205	9.5 *s*
Goldfish, cheese	12	30	2.0 *s*
Graham	2	60	1.5
Melba toast	1	15	.2
Oyster	33	120	3.3
Ritz	3	54	2.9
Rusk	1	42	.9
Rice cake	1	37	—
Rye Crisp	2	50	.2
Saltines	2	26	.6
Sesame, AK MOK	1 oz.	117	2.3
Soda, unsalted tops	10	120	3.2
Triscuits	2	42	1.5
Wheat Thins	4	36	1.4
Zweiback	1	31	.7

The fat content of crackers varies. Beware of saturated fats in the form of palm oil, coconut oil, lard and hydrogenated fats.

GRAIN PRODUCTS

	Amount	Calories	Fat Grams
FLOURS			
Buckwheat	1 cup	333	2.5
Corn	1 cup	431	3.0
Pastry wheat	1 cup	364	.8
Rye, light	1 cup	286	.8
Soy	1 cup	303	14.2 *m*
Wheat	1 cup	400	1.1
Whole wheat	1 cup	400	2.4
GRAINS, MISCELLANEOUS			
Barley	1 cup	696	2.2
Bran, wheat	1 cup	121	2.6
Bran, rice	1 cup	278	12.8
Bulgar	1 cup	602	2.5
Cornmeal	1 cup	421	4.0
Macaroni	1 cup	151	1.0
Millet	1 cup	746	6.8
Noodles, egg	1 cup	200	2.4 *s*
Pasta, whole wheat	4 oz.	400	1.0
Rice, brown	4/5 cup	178	.9
Rice, white	4/5 cup	164	.2
Spaghetti	1 cup	155	.6
Spaghetti w/tomato sauce	8 oz.	179	.5
Stuffing, bread	1/2 cup	198	12.2 *s*
Taco/tostada shell	1	50	2.2
Tortilla, corn	1	67	1.1
flour	1	95	1.8

Most grain products are a good source of polyunsaturated fats.

	Amount	Calories	Fat Grams

SNACKS AND CHIPS

	Amount	Calories	Fat Grams
Cheese puffs, Cheetos	1 oz.	159	10.0
Corn chips	1 oz.	153	8.8
Cracker jacks	1 oz.	114	1.0
Popcorn	1 cup	54	.7
Potato chips	10	113	8.0
Lays	1 oz.	153	9.5
Onion Lays	1 oz.	153	9.5
Pretzels	1 oz.	111	1.0
Tortilla chips, Doritos	1 oz.	139	6.6
Tortilla chips, taco-flavored Doritos	1 oz.	139	6.8

All of the above, except popcorn and pretzels, are fried and contain saturated fats.

MEATS

	Amount	Calories	Fat Grams
BEEF			
Chuck	3½ oz.	327	23.9
Club steak, lean, marble fat	3.3 oz.	260	17.5
lean only	2 oz.	108	4.5
Corned beef, med. fat	3½ oz.	372	30.4
Cubed steak	3½ oz.	261	15.4
Flank steak, lean, marbled	5 oz.	331	14.4
Hamburger, med. fat	3 oz.	224	14.5
lean	3 oz.	140	3.4
Meatballs	1 oz.	78	5.5
Meatloaf	3½ oz.	160	7.6

MEATS

	Amount	Calories	Fat Grams
Porterhouse steak, lean, marbled, broiled	3½ oz.	242	14.7
Porterhouse steak, lean only, broiled	3.8 oz.	204	9.0
Rib roast, lean, marbled	3.7 oz.	264	16.7
Rib steak lean, marbled	3.3 oz.	246	16.0
Rib-eye steak	3½ oz.	440	39.4
Round, bottom, lean, marbled, broiled	4 oz.	271	10.8
bottom only, broiled	3 oz.	205	8.2
Round top, lean & marbled, broiled	3.9 oz.	254	5.9
lean only, broiled	2.8 oz.	173	4.2
Rump, lean, marbled, pot-roasted	2.8 oz.	188	8.7
Sirloin, lean, marbled broiled	3.0 oz.	330	13.8
lean only, broiled	2.7 oz.	128	4.4
ground	3½ oz.	408	34.7
Steak teriyaki	3½ oz.	453	40.3
T bone, lean marbled, broiled	3.4 oz.	235	14.7
lean only, broiled	2. oz.	116	5.4

LAMB

	Amount	Calories	Fat Grams
Arm chop, lean, marbled & fat	3½ oz.	339	27.0
Blade chop, lean, marbled & fat	3½ oz.	340	26.1
Leg, lean, marbled & fat, roasted	3½ oz.	242	14.5
Rib chop, lean, marbled & fat	3½ oz.	423	37.2

	Amount	Calories	Fat Grams
ORGAN MEATS			
Pancreas, beef, med. fat, raw	3½ oz.	283	25.0
Sweetbread, beef (yearling), braised	3½ oz.	320	23.2
Tongue, beef, med. fat, braised	3½ oz.	244	16.7
PORK			
Bacon bits	¼ oz.	20	1.0
Canadian bacon, broiled/fried	1.5 oz.	130	4.2
Cured bacon, broiled/fried crisp	.6 oz.	105	3.1
Ham, fresh, lean, marbled & fat	3½ oz.	306	18.3
fresh, lean only	2.6 oz.	167	4.8
cured butt, lean, marbled & fat	3½ oz.	348	28.0
cured, canned	3 oz.	142	8.5
smoked	3½ oz.	175	11.0
loaf, glazed	3½ oz.	247	14.7
Loin chop, lean, fat	3½ oz.	357	25.6
Picnic, cured, separable lean, roasted	3½ oz.	211	9.9
shoulder, lean, marbled & fat	3½ oz.	312	23.5
Pigs' feet, pickled	1 oz.	56	4.1
Pork, sweet & sour, homemade	7 oz.	386	21.7
Sausage, brown & serve, broiled	1 oz.	118	10.6
canned	3.5 oz.	299	25.9
fresh	1 link	48	4.1

MEATS

	Amount	Calories	Fat Grams
VEAL			
Breast, stewed w/gravy	4 pieces	256	18.6
Cutlet, round, lean, fat	3½ oz.	277	15.0
round, lean only	2½ oz.	194	12.8
breaded	3½ oz.	319	15.0
Loin, med. fat, broiled	3½ oz.	234	13.4
Loin chop, lean & fat	3½ oz.	421	35.9
Veal parmigiana, frozen	7½ oz.	295	14.0
MISCELLANEOUS MEATS			
Frog legs, floured & fried	6 large	418	28.6
Rabbit, stewed	3½ oz.	216	10.1
Venison, roasted	3½ oz.	146	2.2
SANDWICH MEATS, FRANKS			
Bologna, beef	1 oz.	72	6.5
Pork	1 oz.	57	4.6
Turkey	1 slice	60	4.5
Canadian-style bacon	1 slice	40	2.0
Chicken roll, light meat	2 oz.	90	4.2
Corned beef loaf, jellied	1 oz.	46	1.9
Frankfurter, beef	1	145	13.2
chicken	1	116	8.8
Ham, sliced reg. (11% fat)	1 slice	52	3.0
Ham & cheese loaf/roll	1 slice	73	5.7
Headcheese (pork)	1 slice	60	4.5
Italian sausage (pork)	1 link	216	17.2
Kielbasa/Kolbassy (pork & beef)	1 slice	81	7.1
Knackwurst/knockwurst (pork & beef)	1 link	209	18.9

	Amount	Calories	Fat Grams
Lebanon balogna (beef)	1 slice	52	3.4
Liver pâté, chicken, canned	1 oz.	57	3.7
Pepperoni (pork & beef)	1 slice	27	2.4
Polish sausage (pork)	1 oz.	92	8.1
Salami, beef	1 slice	58	4.6
Sandwich spread			
corned beef, canned	½ can	120	10.0
Deviled ham, canned	½ can	220	20.0
liverwurst	½ can	220	19.0
Smoked link sausage, beef	1	130	11.6
pork	1	265	21.6
pork & beef	1	229	20.6
Spam	1 oz.	87	7.4
Turkey, breast	1 slice	23	0.3
Turkey roll, light meat	2 slices	83	4.1
Vienna sausage (beef & pork)	1	45	4.0

Meats, pork products, processed meats and organ meats are all high in saturated fats.

NUTS, SEEDS

	Amount	Calories	Fat Grams
Almonds	12-15	90	8.1
Almonds, roasted	1 oz.	176	16.2
Brazil nuts	4 med.	97	9.9
Cashews	6-8	84	6.0
Chestnuts, fresh	3 small	29	.2
Coconut dried, shredded	2 T	53	3.6
fresh meat	½ oz.	54	5.2

NUTS, SEEDS

	Amount	Calories	Fat Grams
Filberts (hazelnuts)	10-12	97	9.5
Macadamia, roasted	6 med.	109	11.7
Mixed	8-12	94	8.9
Peanuts, raw w/o skin	1 oz.	157	13.2
roasted w/o skin	1 oz.	170	14.0
Peanut butter	1 T	86	7.2
Pecans	12 halves	104	11.0
Walnuts, English	8-15 halves	98	9.7
Pumpkin	1 oz.	155	13.1
Sesame	1 oz.	167	15.5
Sunflower	1 oz.	157	13.2

Nuts and seeds are a source of monounsaturated fats.

POULTRY

	Amount	Calories	Fat Grams
CHICKEN			
Broilers/fryers, light & dark meat w/skin, fried,			
batter-dipped	3½ oz.	289	17.4
w/skin, roasted	3½ oz.	239	13.6
w/o skin, fried	3½ oz.	219	9.1
Broilers/fryers, breast,			
w/skin, fried	½	218	8.7

	Amount	Calories	Fat Grams
w/skin, roasted	1/2	193	7.6
w/o skin, roasted	1/2	142	3.1
Broilers/fryers, drumstick, w/skin, roasted	1	112	5.8
w/o skin, roasted	1	76	2.5
Broilers/fryers, wings w/skin, fried	1	103	7.1
Capon, w/skin, roasted	3 1/2 oz.	229	11.7
Roasters, flesh, w/skin, roasted	3 1/2 oz.	223	13.4
flesh, w/o skin, roasted	3 1/2 oz.	167	6.6
light meat, w/o skin, roasted	3 1/2 oz.	153	4.1
dark meat, w/o skin, roasted	3 1/2 oz.	178	8.8
Chicken roll, light meat	3 1/2 oz.	159	7.4

TURKEY

	Amount	Calories	Fat Grams
Light meat w/o skin, roasted	3 1/2 oz.	157	3.2
Dark meat w/o skin, roasted	3 1/2 oz.	189	7.2
Turkey roll, light meat	3 1/2 oz.	147	7.2
light & dark meat	3 1/2 oz.	149	7.0

OTHER POULTRY

	Amount	Calories	Fat Grams
Duck, w/skin, roasted	3 1/2 oz.	337	28.4
Duck, w/o skin, roasted	3 1/2 oz.	201	11.2
Goose, w/skin, roasted	3 1/2 oz.	305	21.9
Pheasant, w/o skin, raw	3 1/2 oz.	133	3.6

Poultry contains saturated fat, but in lesser quantities than red meat. The saturated fat content of poultry increases with skin.

SALAD DRESSINGS

	Amount	Calories	Fat Grams
REGULAR			
Blue cheese	1 T	77	8.0 *s*
Buttermilk, mix	1 T	58	5.8 *s*
Caesar	1 T	70	7.0 *s*
French	1 T	67	6.4 *s*
Green Goddess	1 T	68	7.0 *s*
Italian	1 T	69	7.1*
Italian, creamy	1 T	52	4.5*
Oil & vinegar	1 T	69	7.5*
Onion, mix	1 T	85	9.2 *s*
Ranch-style, prep. w/mayo.	1 T	54	5.7 *s*
Sweet & sour	1 T	29	trace
Thousand Island	1 T	59	5.6 *s*
LOW-CALORIE			
Blue cheese	1 T	11	0.8
French	1 T	22	0.9
Green Goddess	1 T	27	2.0
Italian	1 T	16	1.5
Mayonnaise-type	1 T	19	1.8
Russian	1 T	23	0.7
Thousand Island	1 T	24	1.6
Vinegar, low sodium, sugar-free	1 T	1	0.0

*Monounsaturated or polyunsaturated depending on type of oil used.

SAUCES, CONDIMENTS, GRAVIES

	Amount	Calories	Fat Grams
SAUCES, CONDIMENTS			
Barbecue sauce	1 T	12	.3
Catsup	1 T	16	.1
Chili sauce, tomato	1 T	16	trace
Enchilada dip	1 oz.	35	1.2
Hollandaise	1/4 cup	180	18.5 s
Horseradish	1 T	7	trace
Mushroom sauce, mix	1/4 pkg.	71	3.2 s
Mustard, yellow	1 T	11	.7
Sour cream sauce, homemade	1/4 cup	124	11.9 s
Soy sauce	1 T	11	—
Spaghetti sauce, canned	1/2 cup	79	3.8
Sweet & sour sauce	1/4 cup	131	.2
Tabasco sauce	1 T	tr.	—
Tartar sauce	1 T	70	7.9 s
Teriyaki sauce	1 T	15	—
White sauce, homemade, med.	2 T	54	4.1 s
Worcestershire sauce	1 T	12	—
GRAVIES			
Beef, canned	1/2 can	77	3.4
Brown, thick, homemade	1/4 cup	164	14.0 s
Brown, mix	1/2 cup	4	.1
Chicken, mix	1/2 cup	41	.9
Mushroom, canned	1/2 cup	75	4.0
Onion, mix	1/2 cup	40	.3

SEAWEED

	Amount	Calories	Fat Grams
Hijiki	100 g.	—	.8
Kelp	100 g.	—	.15
Kombu	100 g.	—	1.1
Nori	100 g.	—	.7
Wakame	100 g.	—	1.5

SOUPS

	Amount	Calories	Fat Grams
Asparagus, cream of	1 cup	87	4.09
Black bean, made w/water	1 cup	116	1.51
Bean w/frankfurters	1 cup	187	6.98
Beef bouillon	1 cup	16	.53
Beef noodle	1 cup	84	3.08
Chicken broth	1 cup	39	1.34
Chicken noodle	1 cup	75	2.45
Clam chowder, Manhattan	1 cup	133	3.4
Clam chowder, New England w/milk	1 cup	163	6.6
Gazpacho	1 cup	57	2.24
Lentil, w/ham	1 cup	140	2.78
Minestrone	1 cup	83	2.51
Mushroom, cream of	1 cup	129	8.97
Onion, w/o cheese	1 cup	57	1.74
Pea, split w/ham	1 cup	189	4.4

	Amount	Calories	Fat Grams
Tomato made w/water	1 cup	86	1.92
Vegetable, vegetarian	1 cup	72	1.93

Cream and meat soups are high in saturated fats.

SUGARS, SYRUPS, JAMS, JELLIES

	Amount	Calories	Fat Grams
Fruit butter	1 T	37	.2
Honey	1 T	61	0.0
Jam, all varieties	1 T	55	.1
Low-cal., all varieties	1 T	29	trace
Jelly, all varieties	1 T	55	trace
Low-cal., all varieties	1 T	27	—
Marmalade, orange	1 T	56	.1
Molasses, light	1 T	50	—
blackstrap	1 T	43	0.0
Preserves, blackberry	1 T	51	trace
Sugar, brown	1 T	52	—
maple	1 T	52	—
white	1 T	46	—

SUGAR SUBSTITUTE
Equal	1 packet	4	0
Sweet 'n Low	1 packet	4	0

SYRUP
Cane	1 T	53	0
Corn	1 T	57	0
Maple	1 T	50	0
Log Cabin	1 oz.	104	0

VEGETABLES AND RAW SALADS

	Amount	Calories	Fat Grams
Alfalfa sprouts, raw	3½ oz.	41	.6
Artichoke, cooked	1 lg.	44	.2
Asparagus, cooked	⅔ cup	20	.2
frozen	⅗ cup	24	.2
Avocado, raw, Calif.	1 med.	306	30.0 *m*
Bamboo shoots	1 cup	36	.4
Bean salad, 3-bean	⅖ cup	75	.2
Beans, canned, Campbell's	7¾ oz.	270	4.0
Chili mex-style, Stokely, Van Camp	1 cup	240	3.0
Homestyle, Van Camp's	8 oz.	270	4.0
in tomato sauce	8 oz.	232	1.8
vegetarian	1 cup	240	.0
Pork & beans, in tomato sauce	1 cup	250	2.0
Beets, raw	2 med.	43	.1
cooked, diced	½ cup	27	.1
canned, sliced	⅗ cup	27	.1
Black-eyed peas, cooked	½ cup	86	.6
canned	½ cup	70	.3
Broccoli, raw	1 stalk	32	.3
cooked	⅔ cup	26	.3
frozen, florets	⅔ cup	27	.2
Brussels sprouts			
cooked	6-8	36	.4
frozen	⅖ cup	37	.3
Cabbage			
Chinese, raw shredded	2¼ cup	14	.1
Green, raw, shredded	1 cup	24	.2

	Amount	Calories	Fat Grams
Green, cooked, shredded	3/5 cup	20	.2
Red, raw, shredded	1 cup	31	.2
Carrot, raw	1 lg.	42	.2
cooked	2/3 cup	31	.2
frozen	3/5 cup	41	.2
Cauliflower, raw	1 cup	27	.2
cooked	7/8 cup	22	.2
frozen	3/5 cup	24	.2
Celery, raw	1 stalk	8	.1
diced	1 cup	17	.1
Chard	3/5 cup	18	.2
Coleslaw	1 cup	173	16.8 s
Corn, white, canned	3/5 cup	60	.3
canned, cream-style	2/5 cup	73	.3
frozen	1/2 cup	88	.9
Corn, yellow, on the cob, cooked	4"	100	1.0
canned	3/5 cup	60	.4
canned, cream-style	2/5 cup	73	.4
frozen	1/2 cup	88	.7
Cucumber, w/skin	1/2 med.	8	.1
Eggplant, cooked, diced	1/2 cup	19	.2
Endive, raw	20 leaves	20	.1
Garbanzo, beans, canned	3 1/2 oz.	179	2.4
Green beans, French-style, frozen	2/5 cup	15	.1
Italian-style, frozen	2/3 cup	37	.1
snap, cooked	1 cup	31	.2
Jerusalem artichoke, raw	4 small	75	.1
Kale, cooked	3/4 cup	28	.7
Kidney beans, red, cooked	2/5 cup	118	.5

VEGETABLES AND RAW SALADS

	Amount	Calories	Fat Grams
Kohlrabi, cooked	2/3 cup	24	.1
Leeks, raw	3-4 med.	52	.3
Lentils, cooked	2/3 cup	106	trace
Lettuce, raw			
Iceberg	3½ oz.	13	.1
Romaine	3½ oz.	18	.3
Lima beans, green, cooked	5/8 cup	111	.5
mature, boiled	3/8 cup	159	.7
Lotus roots, raw	2/3 seg.	69	.1
Mung bean sprouts, raw	3½ oz.	35	.2
Mushrooms, raw	10 small	28	.5
sauteed	4 med.	78	7.4
Mustard greens, raw	3½ oz.	31	.5
cooked	½ cup	23	.4
Okra, frozen	½ cup	26	.2
Onions, raw	1 med.	38	.1
cooked	½ cup	29	.1
Parsley, chopped	1 T	4	trace
Parsnips, cooked	½ cup	66	.5
Peas, raw	3/4 cup	84	.4
cooked	2/3 cup	71	.4
frozen	3/5 cup	81	.5
mature, split, cooked	½ cup	104	.3
Pepper, bell, raw	1 large	22	.2
Pimentos, canned	3 med.	27	.5
Potatoes, baked	1 med.	95	.1
boiled	1 med.	76	.1
fried	½ cup	228	12.1 s
hash-brown	½ cup	229	11.7 s
scalloped, homemade	1 cup	225	9.6 s
Potato salad, homemade	1 cup	363	23.0

	Amount	Calories	Fat Grams
Pumpkin, canned	2/3 cup	33	.3
Radish, red, raw	10 small	17	.1
Rhubarb, frozen, raw	1 cup	29	.2
Rutabaga, diced, cooked	1/2 cup	35	.1
Sauerkraut	1/2 cup	15	.2
Scallion, raw	5 med.	45	.2
Snow peas, frozen	6 oz.	90	.3
Soybean, tofu	3 1/2 oz.	72	4.2
cooked, immature	2/3 cup	118	5.1
fermented miso	3 1/2 oz.	171	4.6
fermented natto	3 1/2 oz.	167	7.2
Spinach, raw	3 1/2 cup	26	.3
cooked	1/2 cup	21	.5
Squash, summer, raw	1/2 cup	19	.1
boiled	1/2 cup	14	.1
Squash, winter, baked	1/2 cup	63	.4
boiled, mashed	2/5 cup	38	.3
Sweet potato			
baked	1 small	141	.5
canned, solid pack	2/5 cup	108	.2
Tomato, raw	1 med.	33	.3
canned, stewed	3 1/2 oz.	27	.1
Tomato paste	1 cup	215	1.0
Tomato puree, canned	29 oz.	321	1.6
Tomato sauce, canned	2/5 cup	31	.3
Turnips, cooked	2/3 cup	23	.2
Turnip greens, cooked	2/3 cup	20	.2
Water chestnuts, canned	16 med.	80	.2
Watercress, raw	10 sprigs	2	trace
Wax (yellow) beans, cooked	2/3 cup	22	.2
Yams, cooked	1 cup	210	.4

MISCELLANEOUS

	Amount	Calories	Fat Grams
Amaranth (red dye)	2 t	4	.1
Bacon bits (imitation)	1 T	33	1.3
Chocolate, baking	1 oz.	185	15.8 *s*
Cocoa, dry	1/3 cup	115	3.6
Gelatin, dry	1 envelope	23	trace
Granola bar	1 bar	109	4.2
Granola fruit bar	1 bar	140	4.0
Olives, black	2 lg.	37	4.0 *m*
Greek	3 med.	67	7.1 *m*
Green	2 med.	15	1.6 *m*
Pickles, dill	1 lg.	11	.2
Kosher	1 lg.	7	.1
Sour	1 lg.	10	.2
Sweet	1 lg.	146	.4
Vinegar	1 T	2	0.0

And did you know? . . . The following items contain no fat!

	Amount	Calories	Fat Grams
Cranberry Cocktail (Ocean Spray)	6 oz.	130	0
Cranrasberry Cocktail (Ocean Spray)	6 oz.	100	0
Frosted Mini Wheats (reg.)	4 biscuits	100	0
Frosted Mini Wheats (bite size)	1/2 cup	110	0
Fruitful Bran	1/2 cup	90	0
Nutri-Grain Wheat	2/3 cup	100	0
Shredded Wheat Squares	1 biscuit	80	0

	Amount	Calories	Fat Grams
Wasa Crackers:			
Light rye	1 slice	25	0
Golden rye	1 slice	35	0
Grits (cooked)	1 cup	125	0
Black beans (cooked)	½ cup	85	0
Boston lettuce	1 outer or 2 inner	<1	0
Chicory lettuce	1 cup chopped or shredded	10	0

6

MENUS FOR LOW-FAT MEALS

MONDAY

	Calories	Fat (grams)
BREAKFAST		
100% bran cereal, 1 oz.	76	1.4
Skim milk, 4 oz.	43	.2
Banana, med.	105	.6
Orange juice, 4 oz.	55	.2
LUNCH		
Turkey sandwich		
3½ oz. white meat turkey	110	1.6
2 slices whole wheat bread	122	2.2
lettuce	2	trace
tomato	8	trace
mustard	11	.7
Apple, 1	81	.5
DINNER		
Spaghetti, 2 cups	310	1.2
Tomato or marinara sauce		
(meatless), 1 cup	65	.6
Grated parmesan cheese, 1 T	33	1.5
Broccoli, steamed, 2 lg. stalks	62	.6
Lettuce, 1 cup	8	trace
Tomato, 1	33	.3
Cucumber, ¼	4	.5
Carrots, ½ cup	22	.1
Oil/vinegar dressing, 1 T	69	7.1
Strawberries, 1 cup	45	.6
TOTALS	1264	19.9

TUESDAY

	Calories	Fat (grams)
BREAKFAST		
Oatmeal, 3/4 cup	108	1.8
Raisins, 1/4 cup	120	.3
Skim milk, 4 oz.	43	.2
LUNCH		
Salmon plate		
6 1/2 oz. canned Atlantic salmon packed in water	237	3.5
Lettuce	4	trace
1/2 med. tomato	16	.15
1/2 carrot	21	.1
1/4 cucumber	4	.5
Lemon wedges	17	.2
Whole wheat roll	90	.1
Oil and Vinegar, 2 T	69	7.1
DINNER		
Melon, 1/2 w/lemon	94	.74
Chicken breast (skinless), broiled, 1 in Dijon mustard	306	6.2
Brown rice, 4/5 cup	178	.9
Steamed vegetables, mixed, 1 cup	31	.2
Frozen yogurt or ice milk, 1/2 cup	92	2.8
TOTALS	1431	24.8

WEDNESDAY

	Calories	Fat (grams)
BREAKFAST		
Grapefruit, 1/2	37	.1
Whole wheat english muffin, 1/2	68	.5
Applebutter, 1 T	37	.2
LUNCH		
Lentil soup, 1 cup	140	2.8
Romaine lettuce, 1 cup	8	.2
Tomato, 1	33	.3
Celery stalk, 1	8	.1
Carrot, 1	42	.2
Cucumber, 1/4	4	.5
Cauliflower, 1/2 cup	14	.1
Olive oil & vinegar, 1 T	69	7.1
Lemon	—	—
Grated parmesan cheese, 1 T	33	1.5
Whole wheat roll, 1	90	.1
DINNER		
Tomato juice, 1 cup	41	.2
Haddock in lemon & white wine, broiled, 7 oz.	300	13.6
Potato, baked, 1	95	.1
Yogurt and chives, 2 T	18	.4
Asparagus, steamed, 2 cups	20	.2
Cauliflower, steamed, 1 cup	27	.2
Popcorn, air-popped, 2 cups	54	.7
TOTALS	1138	29

THURSDAY

	Calories	Fat (grams)
BREAKFAST		
Bran muffin	112	5.1
Applebutter, 2 T	37	.2
Fresh fruit, 1 cup	80	.5
LUNCH		
Chicken breast (white meat)		
skinless, sliced, 1/2	141	3.1
on whole wheat baguette	180	2.0
Lettuce	4	trace
Tomato	8	trace
Dijon mustard	11	trace
Green salad, lettuce	8	trace
mushrooms	14	.2
cucumber	4	.5
tomato	33	.3
lemon, 1/2	8.5	.1
vinegar, 1 T	2	0
DINNER		
Manhattan clam chowder, 1 cup	133	3.4
Swordfish, grilled, 7 oz.	348	12.0
Olive oil & minced garlic, 2 T	79	.9
Carrots, steamed, 1 cup	42	.2
Stringbeans, steamed, 1 cup	31	.2
Sweet potato (baked), 1 small	141	.5
TOTALS	1406	37.2

FRIDAY

	Calories	Fat (grams)
BREAKFAST		
Shredded wheat, 1 oz.	83	.3
Banana, 1/2	50	.3
Skim milk, 3 oz.	86	.4
Grapefruit juice, 4 oz.	48	.15
LUNCH		
Tuna sandwich		
3 oz. tuna packed in water	109	1.6
2 tsp. mayo.	66	7.3
1 large whole wheat pita bread	140	2
Lettuce	4	trace
Tomato	8	trace
Pear	98	.7
DINNER		
Cantaloupe, 1/2 w/lemon	94	.74
Pasta, cooked, 1 cup	155	.6
3 1/2 oz. seafood (fresh shrimp)	91	.8
topped w/1 cup tomato sauce	65	.6
2 T parmesan cheese	66	3.0
Broccoli, steamed, 2/3 cup	26	.3
Spinach, steamed, 1 cup	42	1.0
White wine, 3 1/2 oz.	80	—
TOTALS	1311	19.8

SATURDAY

	Calories	Fat (grams)
BREAKFAST		
Pancakes, plain, 3 med.	210	1.6
Maple syrup, 1 T	50	—
Fresh fruit		
½ banana	52	.3
½ c. strawberries	22	.3
1 small sliced peach	37	.1
Orange juice, 4 oz.	55	.25
LUNCH		
Cheese sandwich		
2 oz. low-fat mozzarella cheese	144	9
2 sl. whole wheat bread	122	2.2
Lettuce	4	trace
Tomato	8	trace
Mustard (Dijon)	11	.7
3-bean salad, ⅔ cup	75	.2
DINNER		
Artichoke, steamed, 1 lg.	44	.2
w/½ fresh lemon	8.5	.1
Chicken breast (skinless), grilled, 1	284	6.2
Corn on cob, 1 small	100	1.0
Green beans, fresh, 1 cup	37	.1
Whole wheat dinner roll, 1	90	.1
Whipped butter or margarine, 1 T	36	3.5
Watermelon, 1 slice	50	.7
TOTALS	1431	26.5

SUNDAY

	Calories	Fat (grams)
BREAKFAST		
Waffles, frozen, 2	190	6.2
Maple syrup, 1 T	50	—
Mixed fruit		
½ c. strawberries	22	.3
½ c. blueberries	42	.3
½ banana	52	.3
LUNCH		
Minestrone soup, 1 cup	127	2.8
Lettuce, 1 cup	8	trace
Tomato, 1	33	.3
Cucumber, ¼	4	.5
Carrot, ½	22	.1
Low-cal Italian dressing, 1 T	16	1.5
Rye crisp cracker, 2 (triple)	50	.2
DINNER		
Hamburger patty, lean, 1	140	3.4
Peas, cooked, ½ cup	104	.3
Carrot, steamed, 1 cup	28	.2
Hamburger roll, 1	114	2.1
Ketchup, 1 T	16	.1
Onions, ¼ cup	15	.05
Mushrooms, 5 small	14	.25
Orange ices, 1 cup	247	—
TOTALS	1292	18.8

7

FAT-BURNING AEROBIC EXERCISE AND WEIGHT-TRAINING VIDEOS

Here is a list of good aerobic exercise and weight-training video tapes. Check the exercise section of your video store and try out a tape before buying it. A thirty or forty-minute low-intensity workout is the most efficient way to burn fat and keep it off without risking injury.

ARNOLD SCHWARZENEGGER'S SHAPE UP WITH ARNOLD
THE BODY SCULPTURE SYSTEM
COSMOPOLITAN AEROBICS LITE
EVERYDAY WITH RICHARD SIMMONS
THE FIRM AEROBIC WORKOUT WITH WEIGHTS, VOLUME THREE
THE GOLD GYM'S PERSONAL TRAINER SERIES
THE JACK LALANNE WAY
JANE FONDA'S COMPLETE WORKOUT
JANE FONDA'S LIGHT AEROBICS AND STRESS REDUCTION PROGRAM
JANE FONDA'S LOW IMPACT AEROBICS WORKOUT
JANE FONDA'S WORKOUT WITH WEIGHTS

JOANIE GREGGAIN'S HIGH ENERGY AEROBICS
KATHY SMITH'S STARTING OUT
KATHY SMITH'S FAT BURNING WORK OUT!
KATHY SMITH'S WINNING WORKOUT
SALSAEROBICS

SOURCES AND RELATED READING

Bailey, Covert. *The Fit-or-Fat Target Diet*. Boston: Houghton Mifflin, 1984.

Bailey, Covert. *The Fit-or-Fat Woman*. Boston: Houghton Mifflin, 1989.

Bennet, William, M.D., and Gurin, Joel. *The Dieter's Dilemma: Eating Less and Weighing More*. New York: Basic Books, Inc., 1982.

Brody, Jane. *Jane Brody's Good Food Book: Living the High-Carbohydrate Way. Forward by Pierre Franey*. New York: W.W. Norton & Company, 1985.

Cluff, Sheila. *Sheila Cluff's Aerobic Body Contouring: The New Low-Impact Exercise Program for the Ageless Body*. Emmaus, Pennsylvania: Rodale Press, 1987.

Connor, Sonja L., and Connor, William E. *The New American Diet*. New York: Simon and Schuster, 1989.

Cooper, Kenneth H., and Cooper, Mildred. *The New Aerobics for Women*. New York: Bantam Books, 1988.

Darden, Ellington, Ph.D. *The Six-Week Fat-to-Muscle Makeover*. New York: Perigee Books, 1990.

Editors, Publications International. *Walking for Health and Fitness*. Lincolnwood, Illinois: Publications International, 1988.

Giller, Robert M., and Matthews, Kathy. *Maximum Metabolism: The Diet Breakthrough for Permanent Weight Loss*. New York: Putnam, 1989.

Gold, Robert, M.D., and Rose-Gold, Kerry. *The Good Fat Diet*. New York: Bantam Books, 1987.

Goor, Ron, M.D., and others. *The Choose to Lose Diet: A Food Lover's Guide to Permanent Weight Loss*. Boston: Houghton Mifflin, 1990.

Heleniak, Edwin, M.D., and Aston, Barbara, M.S. *The Princeton Plan: Put Your Body's "Good Fat" to Work Burning Away Unwanted Fat Forever*. New York: St. Martin's Press, 1990.

Jonas, Steven, and Aronsom, Virginia. *The I Don't Eat (But I Can't Lose) Weight Loss Program*. New York: Rawson Associates, 1989.

Katahn, Martin, Ph.D. *The T-Factor Diet*. New York: W.W. Norton and Company, 1989.

Long, Patricia. *The Nutritional Ages of Women: A Lifetime Guide to Eating Right for Health, Beauty and Well-Being*. New York: Macmillan, 1986.

Peikin, Steven R., M.D. *The Feel Full Diet*. New York: Atheneum, 1987.

Shurtleff, William, and Aoyagi, Akiko. *The Book of Tofu: Food For Mankind*. New York: Ballantine, 1979.

Spodnik, Jean Perry, and Gibbons, Barbara. *The 35-Plus Diet for Women: Kaiser Permanente's Breakthrough Metabolism Diet*. New York: Harper and Row, 1987.

Williams, Xandria. *What's in My Food?: A Book of Nutrients*. Dorset, England: Prism Press; New York: Distributed in the United States by Avery Publishing, 1988.

Winick, Myron, and others, comp. and ed. *The Columbia Encyclopedia of Nutrition*. New York: Putnam's, 1988.